A MODEL FOR GENE THERAPY

A MODEL FOR GENE THERAPY

*Gene Replacement In
The Treatment Of Sickle Cell
Anemia And β Thalassemia*

Ward Merkeley, M.D.

Library of Congress Number: 2005902106
ISBN :   Softcover   1-4134-8940-0

To order additional copies of this book, contact:
Xlibris Corporation
1-888-795-4274
www.Xlibris.com
Orders@Xlibris.com
26865

CONTENTS

Special thanks to Don and Vivian Merkeley,
for the inspiration and imagination;
William Baker,
for the wisdom of liberation;
and Dr. Dana Carroll,
for the guidance.

Introduction

This paper is an attempt to develop a detailed description of a specific application of gene therapy for the treatment of sickle-cell anemia and β thalassemia, both disorders of the β-globin gene. Though this paper is for a specific application of gene therapy, it could serve as a general model for the treatment of several genetic disorders. Always, the underlying question is, how can you get a new gene into a person to correct an otherwise damaging genetic disorder with the least amount of damaging interference?

Overview

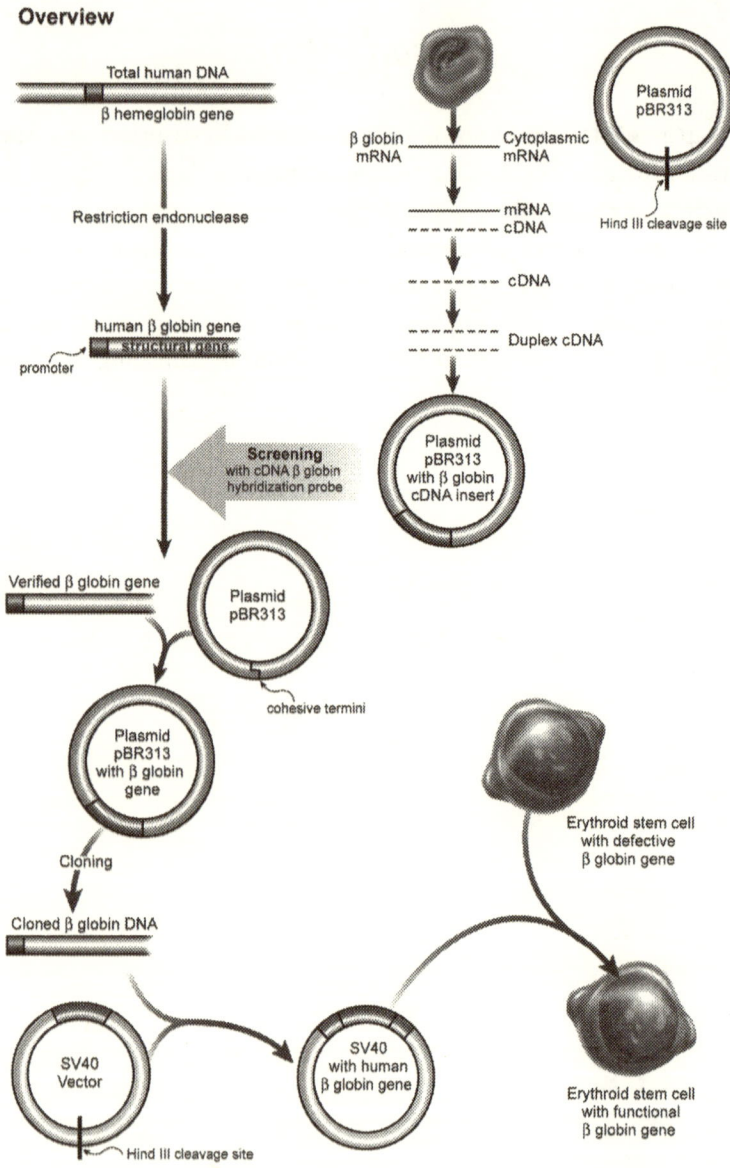

Suggested Criteria for Appropriate Use of Gene Therapy

Before the utilization of gene therapy, it seems the current emphasis should be on prevention of genetic or inborn errors of metabolism. This should involve an exhaustive and comprehensive study of pedigrees: First, establishing whether any member of the family has any known defective genes. If such a circumstance is found, say, known heterozygous sickle-cell anemia, the parents should be encouraged to seek alternative ways of having a family: artificial insemination or adoption. Secondly, a karyotyping of the individual should be done to screen for other genetic defects, which might be reflected as chromosome deletions, translocations and inversion, etc. A more difficult problem to approach and discuss is whether there should be monitoring of fetal development. This could involve detection of a certain number of inborn errors of metabolism, such as enzyme deficiency in muscular dystrophy, Lesch-Nyhan, etc. If an inborn error of metabolism was detected, one could categorize the genetic lesion as to whether or not it would be amenable to therapy after birth. This class of defects would be those in which non-gene-replacement therapy could be initiated after birth, possibly by administration of a hormone, but this approach of replacement therapy would exclude defects in biological molecules, which are necessary for normal fetal development. If one determined that there was a serious genetic defect, then one would have a difficult choice between allowing the pregnancy to go to term or terminate the pregnancy on grounds that the life of the child could be handicapped and, possibly, agonizing. This would be particularly true in those illnesses in which there is progressive deterioration of the individual's life accompanied by mental and physical abnormalities. If one is faced with a certain disease known to cripple and shorten a person's life, on what basis can you decide whether this life is of value? This is a hard question to answer, though I think the science community has an obligation to point out the possibilities and consequences; it ultimately should be a personal choice between the parents; but as much as the desire to have their own child, they should be aware of the consequences for the child, themselves, and society. It would obviously be preferable to correct the genetic deficiency either in the carrier parents before conception or in the affected offspring. Rapid advances in the chemical and biological manipulations of DNA have made it possible to begin thinking how such gene therapy might be approached experimentally. At present, there are many difficulties to be reckoned with of both a technical and a social nature. In this paper, I work through a possible application of the current technology to the specific cases of thalassemia and sickle-cell anemia, both human diseases that have been demonstrated to result from lesions in the globin gene. Inadequacies of available knowledge and procedures are pointed out, and directions for future research and development are suggested.

Genetic Defects in Sickle-Cell Anemia and Thalassemia

General Information

The erythrocytes of a normal adult contains about 97 percent; hemoglobin A (HbA) composed of two pairs of polypeptide chains: two α chains, consisting of 141 amino acids, and two β chains, containing 146 amino acids. The normal hemoglobin is designated therefore as $Hb\alpha^A_2\beta^A_2$ or $Hb\alpha_2\beta_2$. Additionally, there are two other different chains: δ and γ; the latter HbF, $Hb\alpha_2\gamma_2$, is present normally during fetal life and is replaced by HbA progressively after birth. The production of α, β, γ, and δ chains within the erythroid cells is governed by autosomal-allele genetic control. Currently, it is believed that the genes for α and β production are located on separate chromosomes while the control of the synthesis of β, γ, and δ are thought to be located in close proximity to one another on the same chromosome. Each parent contributes one member of the allelic pair of genes; therefore, what determines whether a child is homozygous or heterozygous for a mutant gene are the genotypes of the parents. Hemoglobinopathies refer to hemoglobin disorders that are due to a qualitative difference in hemoglobin production. The heterozygous individual is said to have traits since, as a rule, the trait is harmless; but the homozygous state may have deleterious effects, i.e., sickle-cell anemia, and, therefore, is referred to as a disease. Thalassemia, on the other hand, is thought to be due to the inheritance of a subnormal rate of one or the other of the normal hemoglobin peptides. With the exception of HbC Harlem, only a single amino-acid substitution has been found in each of the abnormal hemoglobin studied (1). Table 1 extracted from *Harrison's Principles of Internal Medicine* classifies the disorders of globin synthesis as either qualitative or quantitative differences:

Table 1

Qualitative abnormalities of the globin peptide (amino-acid substitutions or deletions)

1. Abnormal heme-oxygen interaction

    a. diminished oxygen binding
    b. increased oxygen affinity

2. Normal heme-oxygen interaction

    a. readily precipitating (forms Heinz bodies)
    b. aggregating and interacting (sickles)

Quantitative abnormality of globin peptide synthesis, inherited

1. α chain: α thalassemia (silent, mild, and severe)
2. β chain: β thalassemia

    a. High A_2 β thalassemia (severe, mild, and silent)
    b. $\delta \beta$ (F) thalassemia
    c. Other forms: A_2F thalassemia, etc.
    d. Hemoglobin Lepore syndrome
    e. Hereditary persistence of fetal hemoglobin

3. δ chain: δ thalassemia

This paper will discuss the gene therapy for a qualitative abnormality of the globin peptide-sickle-cell anemia, which is classified as an aggregating and interacting-and, secondly, the gene therapy for a quantitative abnormality of β-globin peptide synthesis, β chain, β thalassemia.

Sickle-Cell Anemia

Definition

Sickle-cell anemia is a chronic hereditary hemolytic disease, which is due to the inheritance from each parent of a gene for HoS. The red corpuscles lack HbA; when they are deprived of oxygen, they assume sickle and other bizarre, but mainly crescentic, shapes (1).

Pathogenesis

The following enumeration extracted from Wintrobe and Haut's discussion of sickle-cell anemia in *Harrison's* will summarize the pathological finding:

1. The sickle cell is a hemoglobin tactoid, thin veiled, and distended by the cell membrane.
2. The homozygous individual's, $HbS\alpha_2\pi^{VAL}_2$, cells sickle in the physiologic range of oxygen tension.
3. Deoxygenation and reduced pH favor sickling
4. Plugs or masses of sickled erythrocytes become solid enough to occlude vessels, and thrombosis and infarction readily follow.
5. A vicious cycle leading to more sickling occurs.
6. Impaired circulation ultimately results in the formation of chronic leg ulcers; infarction; and, later, marked shrinkage of the spleen; hepatomegaly; aseptic necrosis of bone; hematuria; priapism; pulmonary infarction; and central nervous-system complications.

The disease occurs almost exclusively in blacks; and the course is that of a chronic hemolytic anemia (normocytic or macrocytic), which is interrupted by periods of increased weakness, episode of aching pain in the joints, chest pain with ECG changes, or sudden attacks of severe abdominal pain.

Treatment and Prognosis

The following statements are extracted from the discussion of sickle-cell anemia from *Harrison*. No treatment other than symptomatic therapy can be provided. Sickle-cell anemia is ultimately fatal, often before the age of thirty. Death may result from intercurrent infection, renal or cardiac failure, thrombosis, or hemorrhage involving vital tissues, or it may follow one of the abdominal crisis.

Thalassemia

Again, this portion of the paper will draw from extracts taken from Haut and Wintrobe discussion of thalassemia (1).

Definition

The term thalassemia refers to a group of genetically determined diseases caused by partial or complete interference in the synthesis of one of the normal hemoglobin peptide chains. They are characterized by the presence of unusually thin corpuscles, microcytosis, hypochromia, and various degrees of anemia. Its distribution is mainly in those countries bordering the Mediterranean with some Italian communities having reported to have up to 20 percent affliction. Additionally, a high incidence occurs in Thailand and elsewhere in the Far East.

Molecular Lesion

Molecular lesions that produce a deficiency in β-globin synthesis. In general, there are two biochemical varieties of β thalassemia: β^o and β^+ (2). Patients homozygous for β^c defect have the following:

1. No circulating HbA
2. No synthesis of β globin can be demonstrated in their erythrocytes.
3. Variable amount of β-globin $_M$RNA (1-60 percent of normal) in reticulocytes of the patients
4. β-globin gene is intact.
5. Thus, in β^c thalassemia, the molecular lesion appears to preclude translation of β-globin $_M$RNA. The following has been observed in patients with β^+ thalassemia:

    1. A small amount of normal β globin is produced by these patients in the homozygous state.
    2. Quantitative deficiency of β-globin $_M$RNA has been confirmed by hybridization.

3. Several mechanisms have been proposed that could result in
    a decrease accumulation of β-globin $_M$RNA:

    a. Defect may be at the level of transcription of β-
        globin gene,
    b. during processing of the immediate transcriptional
        product to generate cytoplasmic $_M$RNA, or
    c. a decreased stability of the $_M$RNA.

Conversely, in those patients with d β thalassemia and no synthesis of
HbA and HbA$_2\alpha_2\Delta_2$, current evidence indicates that a substantial portion
of the β-globin gene has been deleted, and β-globin $_M$RNA appears to be
absent (2).

Pathogenesis

The primary defect is in the rate of hemoglobin synthesis. There are many
different types of thalassemia, but the majority of cases are when the genetic
anomaly depresses only β-chain synthesis; the disorder is termed β
thalassemia and is expressed in both heterozygous and homozygous forms.
The discussion will be restricted to β thalassemia, for it, like sickle-cell-
anemia disease, involves a defect in the β-globin gene. In the more severe
homozygous state of β thalassemia, there may be nearly complete absence
of HbA, Hbα$_2\beta_2$; for want of β chain and the hemoglobin, which is present
in the hypochromic red corpuscles, is mainly fetal HbF, Hbα$_2\gamma_2$. In β
thalassemia, free β chains accumulate, and these free chains are thought to
exert deleterious effects on the red-cell membrane; and its permeability-
associated with excessive destruction and shortened survival of red-blood
cells, which result in stimulation of erythropoiesis-and causes pronounced
medullary and extramedullary hyperplasia.

Homozygous β thalassemia major (symptomatic) develops insidiously
within the first year or two of life, perhaps starting at birth. Again, the
listing below from *Harrison* (1) will summarize the symptoms and pathology:

1. Marked pallor and great enlargement of the spleen and liver
2. Mongoloid appearance
3. Increase in the medullary portion of the long bones and thinning
    of the cortex

4. Extreme hyperplasia of the bone marrow
5. Anemia is severe, hypochromic, and microcytic.

Treatment and Prognosis

Repeated transfusions have been advocated in β thalassemia major but represent an enormous burden on the patient in terms of risks, especially hepatitis and iron overloading. Prognosis depends on the nature and severity of the inherited disorder. Classic Cooley's anemia-β thalassemia, homozygous-was usually fatal, and those affected often didn't reach adulthood. Less severe forms are compatible with longer life. The heterozygous form may have no influence whatsoever on life span.

Additional Comments

In the case of sickle-cell anemia, with the exception of HbC Harlem, only a single amino-acid substitution has been found in each of the abnormal hemoglobin studied (1). It must be pointed out that both in the case of sickle-cell anemia and β thalassemia, both are essentially normal as heterozygotes.

Preparation of a Plasmid Containing the β-globin cDNA Derived from Human β-globin mRNA

Essentially, the purpose here is to start from β-globin mRNA extracted from the cytoplasm and to synthesize complementary DNA (cDNA) in the duplex form containing as much nucleotide sequence of the β-globin genome as possible. This is just to be used as a probe to help in isolating the gene. The first step is the formation of β-globin duplex cDNA using human β-globin mRNA. How is the β-globin mRNA extracted from the cell? The technique described by Old achieves this (3):

Messenger RNA Isolation

Messenger RNA was purified by affinity chromatography with oligo (DT) cellulose from total polysomal RNA prepared with phenol-chloroform extractions from reticulocytes.

What you have now is a small quantity of β-globin mRNA from which you want to synthesize double-stranded cDNA and eventually incorporate into a bacterial plasmid. Refer to figure 1 to see a review of the steps involved.

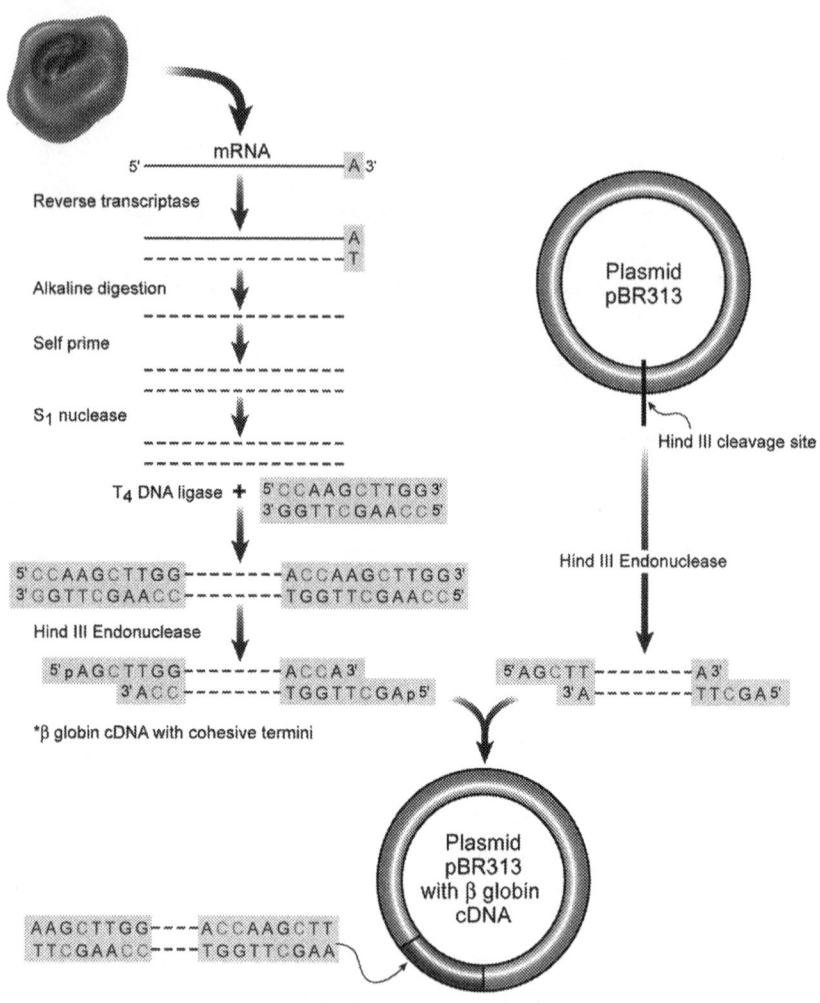

For the purpose of continuity and demonstration, I have selected to use plasmid pBR313 or pBR322 (4). Both have a single *Hin*d 111site in the tetracycline-resistance gene and also conferring-ampicillin resistance. Since the *Hin*d111 site is localized within the promoter for the gene responsible for tetracycline resistance, most bacteria containing a plasmid formed by the insertion of DNA into the *Hin*d111 site are tetracycline sensitive so we can select for ampicillin resistance and tetracycline sensitivity, AMP^R tet^S. If one couples Wilson's method of making double-stranded cDNA with Jeffrey's (5) method of radioactively tagging the new synthetic cDNA by nick translation, we can produce a radioactive hybridization probe. In this simplified description, the single-strand β-globin mRNA is used to make single-strand cDNA by the action of reverse transcriptase (in presence of D actinomycin); then after alkaline hydrolysis, which destroys the mRNA, you have a self-prime reaction using similar condition as in the first step but without D actinomycin. According to Wilson (6), this self-prime reaction results in the conversion of approximately 30 percent of the "full length" single-stranded cDNA into duplex cDNA containing a "hair pin," which can be opened by using single-strand specific nuclease. Finally, the duplex cDNA is isolated by polyacrylamide-gel electrophoresis. Now, in order to insert the β-globin cDNA fragment into plasmid pBR313, which has a *Hin*d111 cleavage site, it is necessary to attach to the β-globin cDNA chemically synthesized restriction-site linkers in the manner in which Goodman does it (7). Refer to figure 1. The example shown here is for the *Hin*d111 decanucleotide, 5'CCAAGCTTGG3'. In summary, the β-globin cDNA fragment has a *Hin*d111 decanucleotide fixed to each end by the action of T_4DNA ligase, and then treatment of the ligation mixtures with *Hin*d111 endonuclease yields duplex cDNA with *Hin*d111 single-stranded cohesive termini. Note in producing the cohesive termini, one must choose a restrictive endonuclease that doesn't cleave the gene.

Next, plasmid pBR313 is cleaved with *Hin*d111 endonuclease, producing a linear plasmid having as well two cohesive termini. Then the linear plasmid DNA is mixed with the double-stranded β-globin cDNA and treated with S_1 nuclease followed by T_4 ligase and E. coli DNA polymerase 1. The ligated DNAs can be used to transform E. coli strains. We can look for colonies containing hybrid DNA molecules by selecting for antibiotic resistance to ampicillin and sensitivity to tetracycline as mentioned above. In Goodman's work on the insulin, they transformed EK2, host E. coli 1776, and transformants were selected by growth on medium containing antibiotics (7). In a similar way, plasmid pBR313, with the attached β-globin cDNA, can be used to transform E. coli 1776, and transformants can be selected by growth on medium containing ampicillin. Only those bacteria that have been transformed by plasmid pBR313 conferring-ampicillin resistance will grow usually. A further cross-check would entail taking a sample from the plaques and streaking them on a medium containing tetracycline to see whether or not they were sensitive because we would expect the transformants to AMP^R tet^S. Further cloning will greatly amplify the quantity of the β-globin genome. The isolated fragments can be subject to base-specific cleavage reactions (7). The cleaved DNA is separated on a 20 percent polyacrylamide gel containing 7M urea and analyzed. Using this method, the nucleotide sequence of the cloned DNA then can be read directly from the gel to verify whether or not it contains β-globin genome-nucleotide sequences. The population of fragments, which contain the β-globin genome sequence, can be used as a radioactive probe after nick translation to help in isolating the β-globin gene from total human DNA.

Isolation of the β-Globin Genome from Total Human DNA

The problem here is, how do you get an intact functional β-globin genome, structural gene, and promoter from total human DNA? The approach described here makes use of the ability of restriction endonucleases to cleave specific nucleotide sequences in DNA. With the appropriate choice of restriction endonucleases, it should be possible to cleave outside the β-globin genome, and, using the techniques of fractionation and screening, determine whether or not we were successful.

A method for the determination of a physical map of restriction-endonuclease cleavage site around the β-globin gene in total human DNA-refer to figure 2.

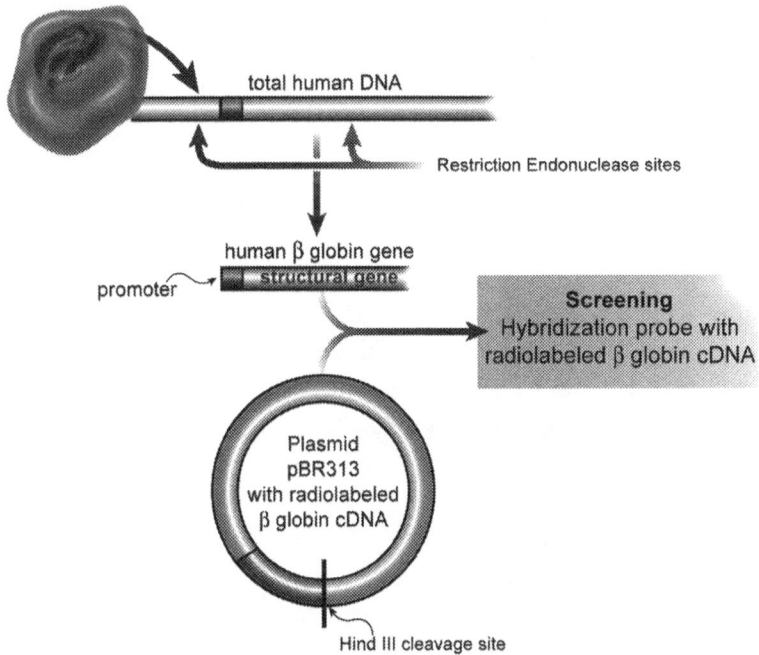

Procedure for the selection of appropriate restriction endonucleases (RE). This could be done by observing the effects REs have on duplex cDNA derived from β-globin mRNA, thus, placing the action of the REs into two classes:

1. REs cleaving within the gene proper or
2. REs cleaving outside of the gene

The next step is to cleave the total human DNA with the appropriate REs, those cleaving outside of the gene, and subsequently isolating the β-globin DNA fragment.

1. Cleaving total human DNA with REs, which will cut outside of the β-globin genome, will result in varying-sized fragments, one population of which will contain the β-globin DNA. Flavell comments that the entire β-globin transcriptional unit and at least some of the sequences involved in regulation of the β-globin gene might well be contained within the kpnI 5.1kb β-globin DNA fragment in the rabbit (8).

2. Then, using gel electrophoresis, we can fractionate by molecular weight the cleaved total human DNA. Knowing the approximate size of the mRNA for the β globin, one can set up a molecular-weight reference to indicate the probable band containing the β-globin DNA fragment.

The use of the plasmid β-globin hybridization to screen initially for DNA sequence of β-globin gene in cleaved fragments

This involves transferring an aliquot of the cleaved DNA fragments to nitrocellulose filters and hybridizing with plasmids containing the β-globin cDNA, which has been previously radiolabelled. Flavell (8) uses such a hybridization technique, which is valuable for our purpose. First, the β-globin genome containing fragments in agarose slab gets is denatured in situ and transferred by blotting at 4°C onto a nitrocellulose filter using a procedure; there, they are blotted dry and baked. The baked filters can be cut into strips and, then after appropriate treatment, can be transferred to an identical solution containing ^{32}P-labelled β-globin cDNA plasmid pBR313. After two days, with the concomitant techniques, the strips are blotted dry and autoradiographed. Since ideally only the hybridization between the radioactive probe and β-globin genome should give a discrete exposure, you have a suitable screening technique. If the plasmid probe hybridizes with a certain aliquot, you can be reasonably sure that this fractionated band contains the human β-globin DNA sequence.

Fractionating the band, initially showing the presence of β-globin gene, would lead to some further purification. Also, the fractionated bands could be further classified by using combination of REs (those that cleave the β-globin genome inside) to make sure it was, in fact, the β-globin genome and not a homologous nucleotide sequence.

The results of these steps should result in a small quantity of human DNA, which, hopefully, contains the β-globin gene. These fragments are going to be longer than cytoplasmic and unprocessed nuclear β-globin mRNA, and it's desirable to be well outside the physical boundaries of the genome on the side of the promoter. The problem now is that you have a small quantity of DNA (probably heterozygous), which must be increased in quantity by amplification technique: cloning.

The techniques in recombinant DNA research are developing now such that given a specific mRNA it will be possible to isolate the gene it originated from.

Cloning of Human β-Globin DNA in Bacterial Plasmid

Up to this stage, we have been successful in cleaving, fractionating, and positively screening for a small quantity of β-globin genome fragments from total human DNA. To increase the quantity of the β-globin genome for subsequent procedures in the experimental protocol, it is necessary to clone the plasmid pBR313 β-globin genome combination, which will result in amplification of the β-globin gene. The method of combining cleaved β-globin genomes to the previously selected vector plasmid pBR313 is identical to the procedure used in the preparation of a plasmid containing the β-globin cDNA derived from human β-globin mRNA. In summary, see figure 3. In order to insert the β-globin genome into plasmid pBR313, which has a *Hin*d111 cleavage site, it is necessary to attach to the β-globin genome chemically synthesized restriction-site linkers. The nucleotide sequence within the synthetic restriction-site linker must be unique and not found in the β-globin genome since if there is a similar cleavage sequence in the β-globin genome, it would cleave the gene. In this case, it would be the *Hin*d111 decanucleotide, 5'CCAAGCTTGG3'. With additional steps, which are covered on page 12, the plasmid pBR313 and β globin are ligated together and used to transform the EK2 E. coli 1776. Transformants can be selected by growth on medium containing ampicillin. Exponentially growing bacteria will replicate plasmid pBR313 β-globin genome DNA. The screening rationale is similar to that described on page 12, where only those bacteria that have been transformed by plasmid BR313-conferring resistance will usually grow. And again, the isolated fragments, which are liberated using *Hin*d111 endonuclease, can be screened using the labelled pBR313 globin cDNA and subject to base-specific cleavage reactions to assure we have the correct nucleotide sequence of the β-globin gene.

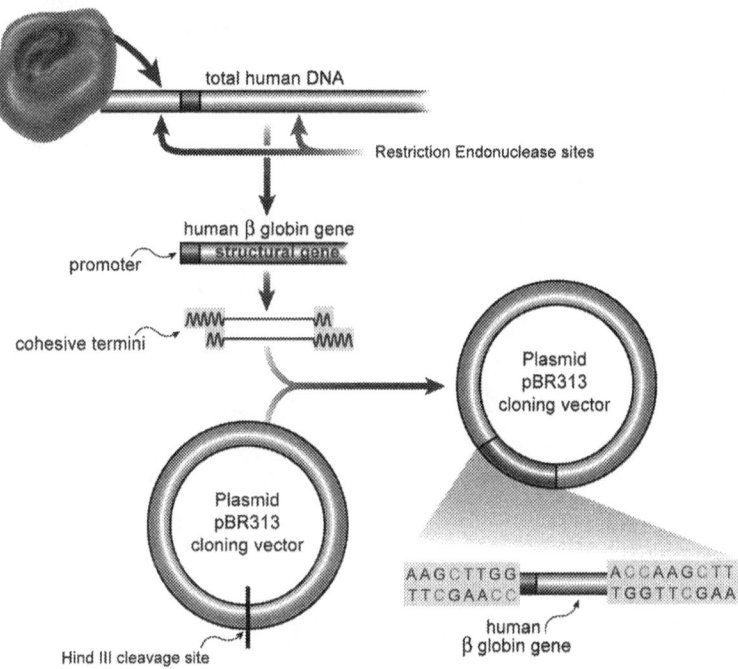

total human DNA

Restriction Endonuclease sites

human β globin gene

promoter

structural gene

cohesive termini

Plasmid pBR313 cloning vector

Plasmid pBR313 cloning vector

Hind III cleavage site

AAGCTTGG   ACCAAGCTT
TTCGAACC   TGGTTCGAA

human
β globin gene

Selection of a Eukaryotic Vector

The eukaryotic vector should be capable of "transporting" the human β-globin gene and transforming mammalian cells, in other words, a vector with the ability of putting the β-globin gene into mammalian chromosomes. One can make a short list of some additional desirable characteristics of a valuable vector:

1. A vector that transforms host cells without cytocidal effects
2. Preferably a vector that transforms but doesn't replicate
3. One that doesn't cause malignant transformation of cells
4. A high-efficiency transforming vector
5. A vector that, once having transformed a cell, has a marker (possibly a detectable antigen), which indicates transformation

Presently, the only cloning vectors utilized in eukaryotic cells have been derivatives of the oncogenic virus-simian virus 40 (SV40) (9)-which contains about five kilobases of double-stranded circular DNA (figure 4).

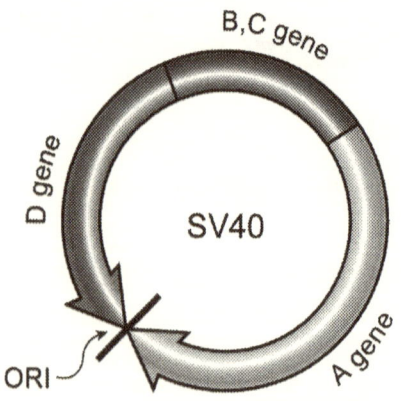

Mutants of SV40 with intact origin (ORT) region and A gene-but defective in the B-, C-, or D-gene regions-can replicate their DNA and transform host cells, but they can only form progeny virus particles with the aid of helper virus, Scott (10). It was discovered that after repeated passage of SV40 stocks at high multiplicity, reiteration mutants occur, Nussbaum (11). Deletions in B-, C-, and D-gene regions of one thousand three hundred base pairs Ganem (12) (from the HpA11 site to the *Eco*RI site) and of two thousand base pairs Goll (13) (from the HpA11 site to the *Bam*11 site) have been replaced by foreign DNAs to produced genomes of over 90 percent of the original length. It is desirable that the SV40 β-globin DNA vector transform the erythroid stem cells without causing malignant transformation of the cells or causing them to be immunologically rejected by the patient due to viral surface antigens. It appears now that transformation is synonymous with malignancy. Hopefully, in the years to come, the elucidation of the SV40 genome structure and function will result in the production of SV40 mutants, which are exclusively able to serve as vectors for inserting genes without malignancy or immunologic rejection-a formidable task.

The next section will discuss the possibility of covalently joining in vitro the β-globin gene to defective reiteration mutants of SV40 DNA segment, which contains the initiation site of SV40 DNA replication, and how later it may be used to transform erythroid stem cells.

Integration of Cloned Human β-Globin DNA into a Modified Eukaryotic Vector SV40

The goal now is to insert cloned human β-globin DNA into a replicating reiteration mutant of SV40. This vector, with the inserted β-globin gene, could then be used to transform, in vitro, erythroid stem cells from patients having sickle-cell anemia or β thalassemia. How do you construct such a vector? The research of Ganem and coworkers (14) is very informative in how to accomplish this task. In summary, they were able to take a 520 base-pair DNA segment excised from bacteriophage λ genome and covalently join it in vitro to an 880 base-pair SV40 DNA segment, which contained the initiative site for SV40 DNA replication. Using wild-type SV40 DNA as a helper, the recombinant molecule was introduced into monkey cells where replication of the λ DNA sequence occurred, and hybrid genomes were encapsitdaded into progeny SV40 virions. The reiteration mutant used was termed d_5 (five tandem repeats of a monomeric DNA segment d_1, 880 base pairs). Each d_1 segment contains one restriction-nuclease cleavage site for endo R. Hpa11 and endo R. Hind111. A 520 base-pair λ DNA segment was prepared by endo R. Hind111 cleavage of the purified EcoRI-B fragments. Now, since both the λ and vector segments have complementary single-stranded termini generated by endo R. Hind111 cleavage, they can be annealed with one another and be covalently closed by ligase (14). As you recall, the cloned human λ-globin DNA produced in the earlier portion of this paper is a 5,100-base DNA fragment having single-stranded cohesive termini created by attaching synthetic decanucleotides having a cleavage site for R. Hind111 (see figure 5).

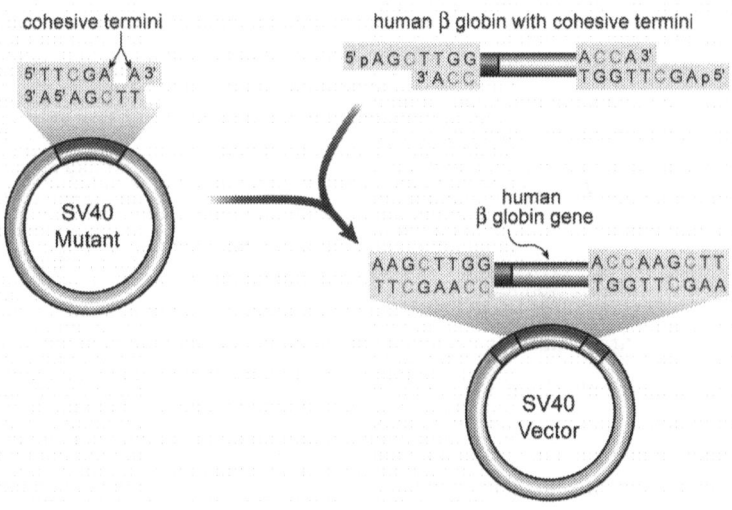

Since both the monomeric DNA segment d_1 (880 base pairs with replication origin) and the cloned β-globin gene have R. *Hind*111 complementary cohesive termini, they should be able to be annealed and ligated. As pointed out earlier, Flavell believes that the five-thousand-one-hundred-base fragment in the rabbit extends beyond the probable boundaries of the β-globin transcriptional unit. And according to Ganem, only segments that are appreciably smaller than SV40 (less than five thousand base pairs) can be successfully used and is, perhaps, the major limitation of using this particular SV40 mutant (*Cell*, vol. 7). In the future, it will be helpful to know the exact size of the human β-globin gene; if too large, then another vector will have to be selected. But can this modified SV40 β-globin gene recombinant transform erythroid stem cells? Before this question is answered, the next section will describe the feasibility of obtaining an erythroid-stem-cell population for transformation.

Isolation of Erythroid Stem Cells

As defined in the criteria, I have decided to limit the discussion in this paper to gene therapy of sickle-cell anemia and β thalassemia to somatic cells and in vitro transformation and, eventually, transplanting the cells back into the patient.

It might be possible to collect over a sufficient period of time by special bone-marrow biopsies a population of erythroid stem cells, which could be maintained and cultivated in a cell-production system. The erythroid stem cells are akin to other primordial cells in that they serve as a reservoir of cells-which, through continued mitoses, give rise to a population of cells-which, after the passage through the erythroid maturation sequences, results in erythrocytes while the stem cells themselves are regenerated. If you isolate an adequate number of erythroid stem cells from the person having sickle-cell anemia or β thalassemia and transform them in vitro, such that the stem cells acquired a new functional β-globin genome, these corrected stem cells could be transplanted back into the affected individual, hoping the autograft would be successful.

At this point, it would be useful to summarize the facts on the stages of development of erythrocytes (see figure 6) extracted from Sandoz's *Atlas of Haematology* (15). As you can see, the pronormoblast, 10-16 μm, is the stem cell of the system, and several comments can be made about the maturation sequence:

1. Immature cells, as a class, are large and become progressively smaller as they are extruded.
2. The nuclear to cytoplasmic ratio decreases as cell matures; nuclei in the older cells are extruded.
3. Cytoplasms of primitive cells are predominantly blue, with Wright's stain, large amounts of RNA; as cytoplasmic structures and secretory products-hemoglobin-are manufactured, the cytoplasm becomes more and more red and less blue.

4. Nuclear chromatic strands of immature cells contain DNA and are eosinophilic while as the nucleus ages, it is more intensely stained, and the color changes from light red to dark blue with Wright's stain.

Proerythroblasts-Round voluminois occupies nearly entire cell.
Nucleus-Fine, dense, uniform, close, meshed chromatic pattern

10-16μm	Pronormoblast-Stem cell of the system Nucleoli-2-5 blue nucleoli Cytoplasm-Deep, clear, uneven blue color
18-22μm	Macropronormoblast
8-16μm	Basophilic Normoblast
8-12μm	Polychromatic Normoblast
8-10μm	Oxyphilic Normoblast I
7-9μm	Oxyphilic Normoblast II
	Pronormocyte (reticulocyte) nonnucleated cytoplasm-Red, showing basophilic stippling
7-8.5μm	Erythrocyte (normocyte)-Mature, final stage of system; a round, flat, biconcave, and nonnucleated disk

The level of intervention in this model of gene therapy is going to be restricted to transformation of somatic cells, erythroid stem cells, in vitro. These erythroid stem cells should probably be collected from the affected individual who has either sickle-cell anemia or β thalassemia since after transformation, by the modified SV40 β-globin DNA, the cells will have to be transplanted back to the donor. Autograft should minimize the immunologic complications that could arise if the donor was different from the recipient. But how are you going to collect a sufficient population of erythroid stem cells needed for transformation and the eventual autograft? Here is one possible approach:

1. Periodically, over several months' biopsy, the patient's bone marrow, after stimulating erythropoiesis, possibly by stimulating with small quantities of erythropoietin

2. After each biopsy using variation of nuclear to cytoplasmic ratio, cell diameter, DNA to RNA content, and progressive accumulation of hemoglobin, devise a method of segregating the cell population by flow-cytometry techniques. Besides, using the morphological facts of the maturation sequences for parameters of sorting cells, the various cell types might be distinguished by supplementary use of vital stains and fluorescent techniques, which don't kill the cells.

3. Having isolated the erythroid stem cells, maintain and cultivate them in a cell-production system, to be covered in next section. Also, one might consider modified cryogenic techniques to store the cells.

A question to be answered is, how many erythroid stem cells are going to be needed to have a successful autograft? Currently, according to Pegg, approximately 10^{10} cells for a 70 kg. man are needed for a bone-marrow transplantation, which is typically 500 ml. of aspirated marrow cells containing all cellular components (Pegg, *Bone Marrow Transplantation*). We are interested in separating the cell population to obtain the erythroid stem cells for transformation. Each of the stem cells, when plaqued in vitro, will give rise to a separate erythroid colony, and Ogawa found that normal bone-marrow specimens varied significantly in their colony-forming capacity, ranging from five to 280 colonies, with an average of about seventy-five colonies per 10^5 nucleated cells (17). Currently, the flow cytometry is capable of sorting 1,000 cells/sec. We can calculate the time it would take to separate the cells 10^{10} marrow cells = 7.5 x 10^6 erythroid stem cells needed 7.5 erythroid stem cell/10^5 marrow cells.

The time needed to sort 10^{10} marrow cells by flow cytometry is 1,000 cells/sec. x 60 sec./min. x 60 min./hr. = 3.6 x 10^6 cells/hr., or 10^{10} marrow cells/3.6 x 10^6 cell/hr. by flow cytometry = 2.7 x 10^3 hrs.

If the magnitude of these calculations is right, it is very discouraging because, using flow cytometry, it would be out of the question. Some other means of isolating the erythroid stem cells must be developed. It might involve sedimentation or immunologic techniques. If this problem cannot be resolved, it may force the level of intervention to the predevelopment stage. The isolation of erythroid stem cells in adequate numbers for transformation and autotransplantation is one of the many technical barriers to evaluate and resolve in this proposed model of gene therapy with its level of intervention and accompanying limitations.

Cell-Production Systems

Methods of obtaining colonies of differentiated hemopoietic cells in vitro, developed over the past few years, have involved use of semisolid agar Bradley (18-19) and Pluznik, methyl cellulose Ichikawa (20), plasma Mcleod and Shreeve (21), liquid continuous flow system Cline and Golde (22) and a few additional means.

For the success of the treatment of sickle-cell anemia and β thalassemia by gene therapy, what is needed is a cell-production system, which would yield a sufficiently large number of cells so they could be transformed in vitro and replanted back into the patient. These papers suggest that large-scale growth of mammalian bone marrow may be feasible, but no such system exists yet. One of the most promising systems is the continuous flow system Cline and Golde (22). It has the following features:

1. Cells grow in suspension chamber modified to permit migration of mature cells, which rest on a 3μ nucleopore membrane.
2. System modified to permit continuous recirculation of external culture medi
3. Bone-marrow cells grown in this system produced mature granulocytes and mononuclear phagocytes. The mature cells could migrate through the nucleopore filter and can be collected in the dialysis compartment. The system permits easy cell retrieval and assessment of cellular differentiation and cytochemistry. It seems probable that an analogous system could be fabricated for the erythroid series as well.

Suggestions for future cell-production systems:

I think it is in the realm of possibilities to achieve a high-yielding cell-production system by using an artificial system, which is analogous to in vivo bone marrow. This would require a thorough characterization of the human bone-marrow morphological architecture and physiology. Besides, serving as a cultivator of future transplanted and transformed erythroid stem cells, such a system could function as a source of transfusionable blood, after suppressing erythropoiesis in the patient, as an alternative to bone-marrow transplantation.

Transformation of Erythroid Stem Cells by SV40 β-globin DNA

Before the actual discussion of how we can detect transformation of erythroid stem cells by the SV40 β-globin DNA, it would be advantageous to describe studies done on in vitro maturation of erythroid cell since it could be a very useful system. The work done by Ogawa (17) and Stephenson on blood-marrow erythropoiesis in culture will form the substance of the following summary. Ogawa found

1. Human-marrow erythrocytes cultured in methylcellulose colony assay technique had a significant degree of maturation synchrony within individual colonies with fluorescamine in order to obtain a ratio of cell-surface labelling to DNA content. This allowed the detection of small numbers of transformants in a predominantly normal population. These are only a few of the imaginable ways of detecting transformation.

For methods forcing transformation, see figure 6.

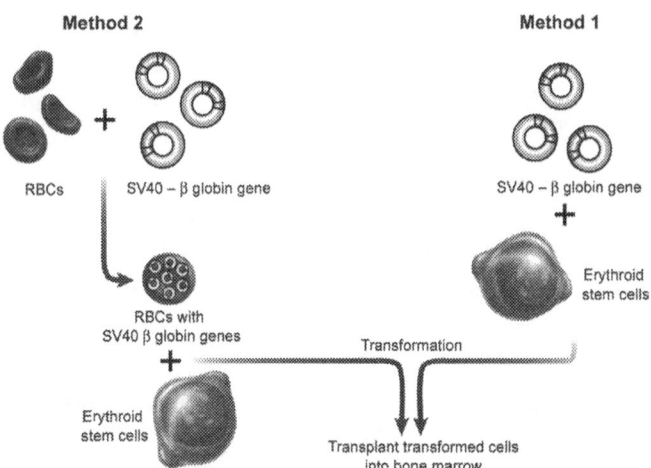

1. The method Ganema used was mixing the recombinant SV40 with African green-monkey kidney cells in the presence of wild-type helper virus. Following this method, one would take the modified SV40 β-globin gene recombinant and mix it in vitro with erythroid stem cells.

2. The second technique would involve placing the modified SV40 β-globin gene into red blood cells during hypotonic hemolysis and fusing them to the erythroid stem cells. This would be an analogous method used by Schlegel to transfer tRNA in culture cell in the presence of Sendai virus (25).

An interesting application for the detection of erythroid stem-cell transformants would be to compare the efficiency of various transformation techniques. One plausible approach would be to do an in vitro analysis of defective erythroid stem cells-ones that make abnormal hemoglobin, which have been submitted to different transformation techniques-and then look for those colonies containing cells with normal hemoglobin. If you find normal hemoglobin-producing colonies, you probably have detected a transformation. A plausible screening method would be to cultivate in vitro the erythroid stem cells, which have previously been exposed to the SV40 β-globin DNA. If these cells were plagued in vitro, it would might be possible to detect an erythroid stem cell that has undergone transformation by the presence of a colony of normal hemoglobin containing daughter cells while the stem cells, which haven't been transformed, would give rise to colonies lacking hemoglobin-containing cells.

Additionally, a recent paper by Hawkes and Bartholomew (24) illustrated that cell-surface labeling, with fluorescamine, indicates the fluorescence of Balb373 A31 cell is considerably decreased after both viral and chemical transformation. This observation, coupled with the technique of flow microfluorometry, enabled nontransformed and transformed cells to be distinguished. As you recall, in the maturation of the erythroid series, there is a progressive disintegration and pyknosis of nucleus. Hawkes and Bartholomew further discuss a second fluorescent probe-propidium iodine, which intercalates into DNA-and is used in combination.

2. The majority of the colonies were small- to medium-sized, fifty-five hundred cells, tightly aggregated, and had a distinct orange

hue due to presence of hemoglobin. Smears of these cells showed polychromatic and oxyphilic normoblasts, 12-17 μ in diameter.

3. A second type of colony was observed composed of large, round, and loosely aggregate cell. There was no evidence of hemoglobin, and the cells failed to stain for pseudoperoxidase with diaminobenzidene and H_2O_2. Smears of these cells showed pronormoblasts and basophilic normoblasts 15-20u in diameter. Also, when these colonies were incubated further over several days, the cells gradually started to accumulate hemoglobin.

4. Nonnucleated erythrocytes, 3-7μ in diameter, were seen within more mature red-cell colonies, though they were extremely hypochromic and microcytic.

5. Colonies did not form in the absence of erythropoietin.

6. Normal bone-marrow specimens varied significantly in their colony-forming capacity, ranging from five to 280 colonies, with an average of about seventy-five colonies per 10^5 nucleated cells.

7. He speculates that immature colonies were derived from colony-forming units analogous to the murine "burst" forming units designated by Axelrod to be progenitors of more mature erythrocytic colony-forming units (23).

We can ask ourselves whether or not Ogawa colony-forming units are, in fact, the erythroid stem cells. If this turns out to be the case, it has some

If the feasibility of transforming the erythroid stem cells by SV40 β-globin DNA is impractical, then attention might be turn to trying to correct the genetic defect before birth. Let us consider one possible situation. Suppose two parents desire to have their own child, but unfortunately, the father was homozygous for a β-globin gene defect while the mother was normal. We have already mentioned the alternative ways of having a family, but let us suppose they decided to have their own child. In such a case, it might be possible to correct the β-globin defect in the father by transforming in vitro his sperm. If we were successful in correcting the genetic defect in the sperm, then the woman could be artificially inseminated. It may turn out that correcting genetic defects in the sperm may be more feasible than in the ovum due to its complexity. But before such an approach can be taken, animal experiments must be done to assess the risks of intervening at such a level.

Autograft of SV40 β-Globin-Transformed Erythroid Cells into Recipient

Assuming up to this point we have been successful in transforming in vitro a previously determined adequate population of the patient's erythroid stem cells, the question to answer now is, how are you going to autograft them? There are the problems of bone-marrow preparation and methods of autografting.

Bone-Marrow Preparation

In all likelihood, you would probably have to eliminate the majority of in vivo erythroid stem cells. This could be done by irradiation of bone-marrow sites. Irradiation, besides the inherent complication, would destroy the other blood-marrow-cell lines; consequently, one may be forced to cultivate other cell lines in vitro, whether they are transformed or not, so when the autograft was done, all elements of the bone marrow would be reconstituted. This is a major obstacle and an inherent limitation of intervening at the postdevelopmental stage.

Methods of Autografting

Currently in bone-marrow transplants, the previous irradiated person receives transfusion of donor bone-marrow biopsies intravenously, and the marrow cells, apparently, migrate to the marrow cavities. For our purpose, this may be one method. Another possibility would be a surgical intervention. Perhaps transfusing the transformed stem cells into the arterial system, immediately vascularizing the bone marrow, injecting the transformed stem cells into the bone-marrow-cavities proper, or putting in a small artificial bone-marrow chamber containing the transformed erythroid stem cells may be successful.

The practicality of autografts is an enormous problem. If it can't be solved, then the treatment of sickle-cell anemia and β thalassemia may necessitate intervention and utilization of gene therapy at an early stage of intervention, say, predevelopment. But as mentioned before, this is a general model, which could be applicable to many genetic disorders. Suppose an adult developed an acquired deficiency of some hormone, e.g., insulin, it's conceivable that one could transform a population of cell by SV40 insulin-gene DNA and place insulin-producing cells in a capsule, which could be implanted in the body, thereby, correcting the deficiency.

Finally, if the autograft of the transformed cells was successful, then there would have to be continuous monitoring of the patient to determine the efficacy of the graft and to detect any abnormal reactions such as malignant transformation or immunologic problem. Needless to say, before gene therapy should be used on humans, the above-presented model of gene therapy must be proven in animal-model studies.

Biohazards

In this particular model for the treatment of sickle-cell anemia and β thalassemia, I have described how the transformed erythroid stem cells originating from the patient would be autografted back to the individual. What problems could possibly arise to endanger the individual? Would taking blood from a person already having hemopoietic problems complicate matters? Would the preparation of the bone marrow for autotransfusion, say, by irradiation, cause irreversible damage? Also, we have no idea whether or not the transformed erythroid stems will assume this natural role once transplanted into the individual or whether or not one transplant will suffice for the rest of the patient's life. Furthermore, we have little knowledge of what the biological character of the transformed cells will be in vivo. Even if we are successful in transplanting erythroid stem having a functional β-globin gene, are these transformed cells going to be malignant or immunologically rejected sooner or later? The only way to begin to answer these questions is by animal-model experimentation.

What controls afford adequate protection against potential hazards of the procedures we have described here? The guidelines concerning recombinant DNA research were issued in 1976 by the National Institutes of Health (NIH). The guidelines were issued to ensure that experimental DNA recombinant will have no ill effects on those engaged in the work, on the general public, or on the environment. They present certain procedures for the containment of recombinant organisms. Containment is defined as physical and biological. Physical containment involves isolation of the experiments. I will only summarize the descriptions here; for more details and elaborations, see the above-mentioned NIH guidelines. Below is a list of physical containments:

> P1-the first physical containment used in most routine bacteriology laboratories.
> P2 and P3-afford increasing isolation while

P4-represents the most extreme measures used for containing virulent pathogens and permits no escape of contaminated air, waste, or untreated material.

According to the NIH guidelines, biological containment is "the use of vectors or hosts that are crippled by mutation so that the recombinant DNA is incapable of surviving under natural conditions. The classification of experiments using the E. coli K-12 containment system has Ek3 as the highest level of containment followed by Ek2 and Ek1. The Ek1 system presently consists of a battery of different vectors and of E. coli K-12 mutants while Ek3 host vectors are Ek2 systems for which the specified containment shown by laboratory tests has been independently confirmed by appropriate tests in animals, including humans or primates, and in other relevant environments.

According to the NIH guidelines, the experiments discussed here using SV40 as a vector containing human β-globin DNA would need the following containment: Such experiments are to be carried out in P3 conditions if the non-SV40 DNA segment is a segment of eukaryotic DNA whose function has been established, which does not code for a toxic product and which has been previously cloned in a prokaryotic host erector system. The use of SV40 would require P3 containment while the experiments using plasmids would necessitate either P3 physical containment and an Ek3 host vector, or P4 physical containment and an Ek2 host vector.

Ethical Considerations

If one wants to employ gene therapy for the treatment of a genetic disorder, what level of intervention is appropriate to correct the genetic lesion? Gene therapy or replacement of defective genes could occur at three levels of intervention: predevelopmental (gametes and zygotes), developmental (embryo or fetus), or postnatal (after birth). When considering gene therapy, one should look from at least two perspectives: a biological perspective and, secondly, a socio-political perspective. Refer to the figure titled "The Continuum of Genetic Intervention." Each one of the perspectives varies according to the level of intervention. From the biological point of view: In group A gene replacement, a newly introduced gene is passed on from generation to generation; hence, it would be new and possibly permanent genetic information. As you move from the bottom toward the top, the genetic efficiency increases, but the results of interfering with development and causing disastrous side effects also increases. So a new beneficial gene replacement could result in an unforeseen congenital defect. In group B, gene therapy at the somatic-cell level with in vitro transformation would not probably be passed on to the next generation, therefore, a self-limiting process. But an in vitro transformation would result in the new genetic information being inherited.

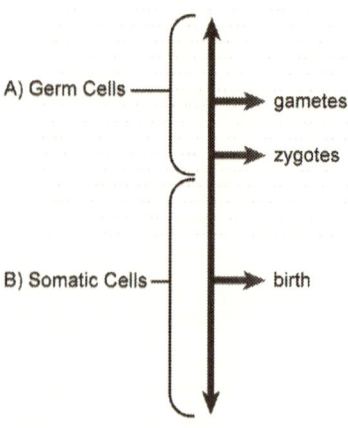

Also, we can divide the gene population into those which are necessary during development (e.g., hormones and induction of target cell-surface receptors) and those genes that could be replaced after development (e.g., sickle-cell anemia and β thalassemia).

I think one of the main considerations in favor of gene therapy is the values of preventive medicine because once a person has a disease due to a genetic disorder, the cost of traditional therapy and medical services is enormous. But an even stronger and greater contribution gene therapy can make is to the well-being of the individual. For a person who has had successful gene therapy, avoiding a crippling disease, has greater potentials in life. Instead of a short agonizing life, an individual can have a more productive and fulfilling life. The evolution of ideas in the scientific community during the last several years has brought us to the concepts of recombinant DNA and its application. The scientific community is acutely aware of some of the obvious ramifications of genetic engineering. For as scientists further understand the biological truths and how to use them, people have an increased control of their destiny, good or bad. Therefore, as before, the beneficial uses and damaging results of genetic engineering depend upon the attitudes and decisions of mankind.

Problems of Recombinant DNA Techniques

Recombinant DNA is a sophisticated means of biological intervention, and it entails developing complex techniques to achieve it. It will be a very powerful experimental and technical tool in biology, but one has to wonder how it will change our lives. What are we heading for? Recombinant DNA is an incredible exploratory tool. In as much as the light and electron microscopes gave us a view of biology never seen and understood before, so will research inrecombinant DNA begin to unravel the complexities of the gene, chromosomes, and the corresponding regulation and function of each. Recombinant DNA research is the frontier of biology now but still at the periphery of elucidating biological questions, which will be the core of understanding. What are some of the possible discoveries we can anticipate developing from recombinant DNA research? In the section titled "Isolation of the Globin Gene from Total Human DNA," such technique has generalized implications. One day it is conceivable that a large percentage of genes will be localized to specific chromosomes. Such genetic mapping might shed light upon the possible affects of gene arrangement. Questions such as what influence does one gene have upon another neighboring gene might be answered. Also, it would be interesting to know what are the consequences of a gene being located, say, adjacent to the centromere as opposed to at the end of a chromosome in terms of mitoses and meiosis and events such as translocation, deletion, inversion, etc. Such knowledge would be invaluable in terms of chromosomes analysis and being able to detect genetic errors.

The section titled "Integration of Cloned Human β-Globin DNA into a Modified SV40 Erkaryotic Vector" and "Transformation of Erythroid Stem Cells by SV40 β-Globin DNA" are techniques that, when developed, could have many uses. It is essentially a means of inserting any new genetic information into DNA. Depending on the size limitation, it is conceivable that one to several genes may be integrated into the recipient's chromosomes. With new genetic information, the living organisms could take on new properties. Bacteria have already been designed, which have the ability to produce synthetic hormone, e.g., somatostatin. In the years to come, one can see many other ways to use microorganism to produce biological molecules. It is also conceivable that the known pathogen in bacteria and viruses may be eradicated by manipulation involving inserting new genetic information into them, which changes them to innocuous mutants that have also a conditional lethal mutation to some circumstance of choice. But the real problem to be concerned about would be manipulation involving humans. Would it be right to give humans new genetic information? What does that mean in terms of mankind?

There are two additional aspects to the ethical considerations: First, is it ethical to subject individuals or populations to potential dangers of this type of intervention? The danger and safety of using gene therapy are two aspects that need to be dealt with. On paper, the techniques necessary for gene therapy can be developed logically, successively, orderly, and with the utmost scrutiny. As much as we can predict success on theoretical grounds, in reality, the actual achievement is a series of many hurdles, which must be dealt with. No matter if we succeed in 99 percent of the project, one missed technical hurdle, and the patient loses. Gene therapy would be a series of technical procedures each one distinctly different, and undetected error would be carried through the remainder of the procedures. In medical therapeutic procedure, errors are made, which are hopefully correctable, thus, restoring the integrity of individual. But how can we now guarantee the safety of gene therapy? We cannot. It will be experimental and should first be worked through animal models. There is an enormous amount of groundwork, which needs to be done before gene therapy, in any sense of the word, can be considered feasible. Maybe in the years to come, the feasibility and risks of gene therapy will be better understood. Then the potential dangers of the type of intervention can be predicted. Once this level of knowledge is reached, some of the risks and benefits of a particular gene-therapy intervention can be pointed out to the individual.

The second consideration is, is it ethical to withhold potential benefits when the technology to provide them is, or can, soon be made available? The answer to this question is dependent upon the answers given in the last paragraph in part. If you could realistically appraise the risks and benefit of gene therapy and determine that the potential benefits exceed the potential risks, then it would be unethical to withhold potential therapeutic intervention as much as it would be unethical to withhold, say, an antibiotic, an emergency surgical procedure, or any other life-saving medical intervention. But on the other hand, if the potential risks and benefits were unclear, then it would be wise to hold back. The ethical considerations of any medical knowledge and its application are difficult. History shows instances of success and failure. How did Jenner, Fleming, or Einstein view their contributions experimentally and retrospecting? How can we avoid disasters such as the delcon shield, the unforeseen effects of diethylstilbestrol, or the consequences of massive thymus-irradiation programs?

Finally, if gene therapy becomes feasible, who will decide who receives it, and who will decide what are its limitations? Recombinant DNA research is an enormously expensive undertaking. The groups of people who have the monies for research will direct the development of recombinant DNA research and its application. Two apparent sources of funds are the government and private industries. The government can control research by setting up guidelines for recombinant DNA research such as the National Institutes of Health did in 1976. The guidelines were sent to approximately twenty-five thousand NIH grantees and contractors. Initially, it was the scientist doing recombinant DNA research who called for a moratorium on certain kinds of experiments in order to assess the risks and devise appropriate guidelines. I believe a national, as well as international, committee setting up guidelines and monitoring recombinant DNA research would be in the best interest and service of mankind. But how much is needed short of impinging upon the right of scientific inquiry?

I definitely feel the guidelines established by the National Institutes of Health are headed in the right direction. Eventually, consideration will have to be given to who should receive gene therapy. Guidelines in this concern will need to be set up. Whatever they will be is open for discussions. This consideration will be akin to the decision process concerning who should go on a kidney machine, or have an organ transplant or a coronary bypass.

As advances occur in recombinant DNA research, the question always to be asked is, in what direction should we go, and what should we not do? What will be the limitations in gene therapy?

Finally, genetic intervention is a very large step, and it is difficult to predict confidently the full ramifications of any particular alteration particularly with our limited knowledge at present; but even as our understanding of short-term biological processes improve, it will be difficult to predict long-term effects. A striking example of this is the evolutionary process; it has been time-tested over millions of years, and it works. Living things follow fundamental biological rules, which are operating continuously whether we perceive them or whether we will possibly never understand them. Nature is a balance between biological systems. Changing one element in the system has ramifications for the other dependent members. Man is beginning to realize the powerfulness but subtle balance, which occurs in nature, and how abuse can result in disastrous ecological consequences. We are all in it together. Recombinant DNA knowledge and application are at the heart of the evolutionary process. It is control, and frankly, the possibilities are both promising and frightening. When you start doing genetic manipulations, even if they are of good intention, and shift the genetic balance, I don't think anybody can know what the new balance will be. Certainly, we can predict, but it's crucial that we be humble and admit that even though we know some of the truths, it is probably little compared to the whole. This makes the current decision concerning recombinant DNA an enormous responsibility, which should proceed with great deliberation and caution.

References

1. *Harrison's Principles of Internal Medicine*, 7th ed. (1974)
2. *P.N.S.A.* vol. 74, no. 9 pp3960, September (1977)
3. *Cell*, vol. 8, 13-18, May (1976)
4. *J. Gen. Microbiol* 86(1): p. 111 Jan.(1975)
5. 611, vol. 8, 429-439, October (1977)
6. *Science*, vol. 196, 202, April (1977)
7. *Science*, vol. 196, 1313, June (1977)
8. *Cell*, vol. 12, p. 429, Oct. (1977)
9. Kelly, T. J. Jr., Nathans, D. *Adv. Virus Res.*, vol. 21. (1976)
10. Scott, W. A., Brockman, W.W., Nathans, D. *Virology* 75:319 (1976)
11. Nussbaum, A. L., *INSA*, 73: 1068 (1976)
12. Hamer, D. H., Davoli, Thomas, Fareed, G. C. *J. Mol. Bio. (1977)*
13. Goff, S., Berg, 1976. *Cell* 9:695 (1976)
14. *Cell* vol. 7, p. 349 March (1976)
15. *Sandoz Atlas of Haematology*, 2nd ed. 51, (1973)
16. *Bone marrow transplantation*, D. E. Pegg, Lloyd-Luke LTD, (1966)
17. *Blood*, vol. 48, no. 3 (September), 1976
18. *Aust. J. Exp. Biol. M. Sci*, 44, 287 (1966)
19. *J. cell. Comp. Phusiol.*, 66, abd *Exp. Cell* Res., 43, 553 (1965)
20. *Proc. Acad. Sci*, USA, 56, 488 (1966)
21. Mcleod and Shreeve (1971)
22. *Blood*, vol. 47, no. 3 March, (1976)
23. *Hemopoiesis in Culture*. Washington, D.C., US Gov., Printing Office, (1974)
24. *PNAS*. vol. 74, no. 4, p.1626, April (1977)
25. *ICN-UCLA Symposia on Molecular and Cellular Biology*, vol. 5, 1976

February 7, 1978

Report on the independent study program of Ward Merkeley, autumn quarter 1977 (Microbiology 796).

Letter from: Dr. Dana Carroll

Ward Merkeley came to me early in the autumn quarter, 1977, expressing an interest in recombinant DNA. I agreed to sponsor him in an independent study project on this subject. Because of his interest in the medical perspectives for recombinant DNA, we agreed it would be most sensible for him to do library research and write a paper on the feasibility of using recombinant DNA techniques, in conjunction with other procedures, in an example of gene therapy. After much searching (by him) of the literature in medical genetics, we decided to focus on two genetic defects affecting the human b-globin gene: sickle-cell anemia and b thalassemia. Using published procedure-developed for globin mRNAs and genes, in some cases, and for other purposes in others-Ward developed a highly credible scheme for isolation and amplification of the human b-globin gene. He then speculated, on the basis of available facts, on how one might transfer this gene in a functional state to an afflicted individual. He included in his paper a discussion of the biohazards associated with the proposed procedures and the ethical considerations surrounding genetic manipulation of humans.

In the finished product, Ward has done an excellent job of bringing together all the aspects of his proposal, from molecular biology to clinical medicine. Despite our efforts to limit it where possible, the scope of this undertaking is very broad. Throughout, I have been impressed by Ward's application of his resources to develop an understanding of each of the many aspects of the problem and his ability to come to grips with the central difficulties. He was unfamiliar with the relevant details of modern molecular biological dogma but mastered these sufficiently to make sensible proposals concerning RNA and DNA isolation and analysis, preparation and cloning of recombinant DNAs, viral transformation, and several aspects of cell biology. These he learned with my guidance, but in addition and on his own initiative, he investigated current methods in bone-marrow transplant and tissue culture since these were necessary to the final stages of his proposal. The safety and ethical considerations are a bit more nebulous and further afield, but these, too, he took seriously. Though not unflawed, his paper is most impressive, considering its scope and the limited amount of time he had to work on it. I plan to enlist his help in presentation of the subject of recombinant DNA technology to a Continuing Medical Education class this spring.

Ward and I have discussed the possibility of his working in my laboratory on some aspect of recombinant DNA research. Naturally, we cannot begin to undertake the practical realization of the scheme he proposed in his paper. Nonetheless, if it ultimately suits his schedule and desires, I would gladly accept him as a coworker. He has a genuine interest and aptitude for which I am happy to provide scope and encouragement.

Dr. Dana Carroll